The Rebellion Of Glucose

Innovatory Oblige in Adapting to your glucose

By

Julian T.Chapman

Table of Contents

INTRODUCTION

Glucose is vital to energy utilization. Carbs, lipids, and proteins all eventually separate into glucose, which then fills in as the essential metabolic fuel of warm-blooded creatures and the general fuel of the hatchling. It fills in as the significant antecedent for the union of various carbs like glycogen, ribose, deoxyribose, galactose, glycolipids, glycoproteins, and proteoglycans. In actuality, in plants, glucose is blended from carbon dioxide and water (photosynthesis) and put away as starch. At the cell level, most frequently, glucose is the last substrate that enters the tissue cells and converts to ATP (adenosine triphosphate).

ATP is the energy money of the body and is consumed in more than one way including the dynamic vehicle of atoms across cell layers, withdrawal of muscles and execution of mechanical work, engineered responses that assist to make chemicals, cell films, and other fundamental particles, nerve drive conduction, cell division and development, and other physiologic capabilities...

Chapter 1

What is Glucose

There is a wide range of types and types of caloric sugars that are by and large called "sugar." The most natural sort of sugar is table sugar. Experimentally talking, table sugar is sucrose, a disaccharide made of equivalent pieces of two monosaccharides: fructose and glucose.

Monosaccharides are single units of sugar and are frequently alluded to as "straightforward" sugars. The three fundamental monosaccharides that we consume are fructose, galactose, and glucose. They join in different matches to shape the three sorts of disaccharides (two connected sugar units) that are most significant in human sustenance: lactose, maltose, and sucrose.

Glucose is the consistent idea in each of these. It is important for sucrose (connected with fructose), lactose (connected with galactose), and maltose, which comprise two connected glucose units.

Notwithstanding glucose being vital to disaccharides, it is likewise a basic piece of life.

Glucose is our body's primary wellspring of energy, for certain tissues like the cerebrum require a consistent inventory. Glucose is alluded to as "glucose" since it circles in our circulatory system as a wellspring of promptly accessible energy. It is likewise put away in the body as glycogen for energy savings during times when adequate glucose may not be free in the blood.

Where is the source of glucose?

Glucose is the most widely recognized monosaccharide tracked down in nature. In plants, it is produced through photosynthesis. A few plants store glucose in connected chains. Starch is the name of these chains.

Normal starch-containing food varieties incorporate corn, potatoes, rice, and wheat. Starch is monetarily isolated from these entire food sources to make dextrose, glucose, maltodextrins, polyols, and high fructose corn syrup to be utilized as fixings in the development of certain food sources, refreshments, dressings, and sauces.

Glucose monosaccharides (not as a feature of starch) are likewise tracked down normally in certain food varieties. The most focused entire food wellspring of glucose monosaccharides is honey, trailed by dried natural products like dates, apricots, raisins, currants, cranberries, prunes, and figs.

Is glucose a characteristic or added sugar?

The sugar that we consume is much of the time depicted as normal sugar or added sugar, contingent upon its source. Glucose is viewed as a characteristic sugar when eaten straightforwardly from entire food varieties like apricots and dates.

Glucose is viewed as an additional sugar when eaten from bundled food sources and refreshments to which it has been added during assembling. Tragically, somewhere around one out of ten American grown-ups eats the suggested measure of natural products or vegetables each day, while six of every ten American grown-ups eat more added sugars than is suggested.

How is glucose processed?

Glucose doesn't need processing. All things being equal, it is caught up in the small digestive tract straightforwardly into the circulation system, where it very well may be utilized for energy or at last put away as glycogen in muscle and liver. We consume glucose straightforwardly from food varieties like honey, and we additionally get glucose from food sources and refreshments that contain lactose, sucrose, and starch. At the point when we eat starch-containing

food varieties, the spit in our mouth should initially separate starch into maltose (sets of connected glucose units). Maltose is then separated further into its singular glucose units, making them accessible for ingestion. Like maltose assimilation, when we consume lactose and sucrose, glucose is retained after being isolated from its accomplice monosaccharide (galactose in lactose and fructose in sucrose).

The means engaged with disaccharide and starch processing makes it take more time to retain glucose, which results in to a lesser degree an ascent in glucose than consuming glucose straightforwardly.

Could our bodies at any point make glucose?

Our bodies expect glucose to work. It is especially basic for our cerebrum, as this organ utilizes around 60% of the glucose that our bodies use. Be that as it may, glucose doesn't necessarily in all cases need to come quickly from food varieties and refreshments. Glucose is created by the body to guarantee that we generally have the sum required. One way this is done is by separating down glycogen to free the glucose it contains. Glycogen breakdown happens between dinners or during times of extremely active work.

The body can likewise deliver glucose through gluconeogenesis, a cycle by which the body (fundamentally the liver) makes glucose from non-carb sources. Gluconeogenesis happens when glycogen stores become low and glucose utilization is excessively low or nonexistent, for example, during times of starvation or delayed fasting.

What is DIABETES

Diabetes is an infection that influences your body's capacity to create or utilize insulin. Insulin is a chemical. At the point when your body transforms the food you eat into energy (likewise called sugar or glucose), insulin is delivered to assist with moving this energy to the phones. Insulin goes about as a "key." the synthetic message advises the cell to open and get glucose. Assuming you produce practically no insulin or are insulin safe, an excess of sugar stays in your blood. Blood glucose levels are higher than typical for people with diabetes. There are two primary kinds of diabetes: Type 1 and Type 2.

What is Type 1 diabetes?

At the point when you are impacted with Type 1 diabetes, your pancreas doesn't create insulin. Type 1 diabetes, when called adolescent diabetes, is many times analyzed in kids or teenagers. Notwithstanding, it can likewise happen in grown-ups. This type represents 5-10 percent of individuals with diabetes.

What is Type 2 diabetes?

Type 2 diabetes happens when the body doesn't create sufficient insulin, or when the phones can't utilize insulin appropriately, which is called insulin opposition. Type 2 diabetes is regularly called "grown-up beginning diabetes" since it is analyzed sometime down the road, for the most part after the age of 45. It represents 90-95 percent of individuals with diabetes. As of late, Type 2 diabetes has been analyzed in more youthful individuals, including kids, more regularly than previously.

Are there different types of diabetes?

Gestational diabetes happens during pregnancy and influences around 18% of all pregnancies, as per the American Diabetes Affiliation. Gestational diabetes as a rule disappears after pregnancy, yet whenever you've had gestational diabetes, your odds are higher that it

will occur in later pregnancies. In certain ladies, pregnancy reveals Type 1 or Type 2 diabetes and these ladies should proceed with diabetes treatment after pregnancy. There is by all accounts a connection between the propensity to have gestational diabetes and

Type 2 diabetes, and numerous ladies who had gestational diabetes fostered Sort 2 diabetes later on. Gestational diabetes and Type 2 diabetes both include insulin obstruction. Certain essential way-of-life changes might assist with forestalling diabetes after gestational diabetes.

Another structure is prediabetes. This condition causes an individual's glucose levels to be higher than typical but not sufficiently high to be determined to have diabetes. The American Diabetes Affiliation assesses that there are 84.1 million Americans that have pre-diabetes notwithstanding the 30.3 million with diabetes.

What causes diabetes?

Hereditary qualities, way of life, and climate can be reasons for diabetes. Eating an undesirable eating regimen, being overweight or stout, and not practicing enough might assume a part in creating diabetes, especially Type 2 diabetes. Type 1 diabetes is brought about by an immune system reaction. The body's resistant framework assaults and obliterates the insulin-creating beta cells in the pancreas.

How does diabetes influence my body?

Over the long run, high glucose levels (additionally called hyperglycemia) can prompt kidney sickness, coronary illness, and visual deficiency. The abundance of sugar in the circulation system can harm the small veins in your eyes and kidneys and can solidify or limit your conduits.

What are the side effects of diabetes?

Outrageous thirst Continuous pee
Foggy vision Outrageous yearning Expanded
sluggishness
Strange weight reduction

How might I see whether I have diabetes?

Some of the time a normal test by an eye specialist or foot specialist will uncover diabetes. Diabetes influences the flow to your feet and the little veins in your eyes. On the off chance that your eye specialist or your foot specialist suspects you have diabetes, they will suggest you see your standard doctor for a glucose level test.

The most well-known test is a fasting blood glucose test. After not eating for something like eight hours, normally short-term, your PCP will take a blood test. The typical, non-diabetic reach for fasting blood glucose is 70 to 110 mg/dl. Assuming your level is 126 mg/dl or more noteworthy, you might have diabetes.

Chapter 2

Why are Glucose spikes Terrible for us

Blood sugar spikes can be harmful to our health because they can lead to a condition known as hyperglycemia. When our body breaks down food, it releases sugar into our bloodstream. This triggers the pancreas to produce insulin, which helps to regulate our blood sugar levels.

However, when we consume foods that are high in sugar and simple carbohydrates, our blood sugar levels can rise too quickly, causing a spike in insulin production. This sudden increase in insulin can cause our blood sugar levels to drop rapidly, leading to symptoms such as dizziness, fatigue, and headaches.

Over time, repeated blood sugar spikes can increase our risk of developing insulin resistance, a condition in which our cells become less responsive to insulin. This can lead to type 2 diabetes, a chronic condition that can cause a range of complications, including nerve damage, kidney disease, and cardiovascular disease. To avoid blood sugar spikes, it is important to eat a balanced diet that includes complex carbohydrates, fiber, and protein, and to avoid foods that are high in added sugars and refined carbohydrates. Regular exercise can also help to regulate blood sugar levels and improve insulin sensitivity.

High glucose levels are generally connected with type 2 diabetes however truth be told, normal glucose spikes can have a wide-arriving at influence across our whole body. Despite some short-and long haul impacts of predictable glucose spikes, there's uplifting news limiting the spike, and the accident can go far to causing you to feel great and well.

Glucose is the fundamental sort of sugar in the blood and without it, we would stop existing. It's the body's favored energy source and keeps everything working regularly. There can, in any case, be an overdose of

something that is otherwise good, and an excess of glucose can hurt us — frequently without us understanding it. All in all, what is a glucose spike? Also, what's the significance here for your well-being? A glucose spike happens when glucose develops in the circulation system and glucose levels increment.

We will generally relate raised glucose levels with conditions like sort 2 diabetes and keep in mind that that is unquestionably right, an amazing 80% of individuals without diabetes additionally experience high glucose spikes.

This most frequently occurs after eating, when the food we eat is separated during processing. Furthermore, it's not only the sweet stuff that you want to watch out for — all carbs separate into glucose, which then, at that point, enters the circulation system.

We will quite often ingest more glucose than we want, which causes glucose levels to rise quickly and this causes a spike. To redress, our body delivers more insulin to assist with bringing down glucose levels. This can once in a while make levels plunge excessively low thus starting the unfortunate rollercoaster of ups and downs in glucose levels.

We ought to make it clear at this stage that glucose spikes are typical whether or not you have type 2 diabetes or not — particularly after eating a high-carb feast. A solitary spike won't prompt long haul confusions like sort 2 diabetes, however, can in any case bring about transient medical problems.

As the blood moves around the body, glucose is conveyed to cells where it's transformed into energy. This energy is utilized to control each and everything that occurs in our bodies.

That is the basic form of occasions however there's a heap more going on. It's nothing excessively muddled except that we believe it's a very intriguing understanding of what rehashed glucose spikes truly mean,

We enter a condition of oxidative pressure, Everything begins with something many refer to as mitochondria, which are tracked down in practically every phone in the body. While minute in size, they're significant because it's here that glucose is transformed into the energy that drives the cell. Mitochondria generally just consume as the need might arise for energy yet when we have a glucose spike, we're sending a lot of glucose to our cells excessively fast, basically suffocating our mitochondria in glucose.

Ongoing logical hypothesis recommends that when our mitochondria are suffocating in glucose, our phones discharge minuscule particles called free extremists. Despite their fairly certain name, free extremists are something perilous to have drifting around because they can harm anything they come into contact with. Our bodies can manage them with some restraint however when there are too many, they become unmanageable. With rehashed glucose spikes, the amount of free extremists created is excessive and our body ultimately enters a condition of oxidative pressure.

Oxidative pressure isn't generally hurtful however uncontrolled oxidative pressure in the long haul adds to various circumstances like coronary illness, mental degradation, and type 2 diabetes.

Glucose chances upon different atoms in the body — and harms them, At the point when we toast bread, we spread the word about it brown — this is the Maillard response and it happens when a glucose particle chances upon one more sort of particle, which causes a response. The subsequent article then said

to have been 'glycated' and when this occurs, it's harmed until the end of time.
This interaction doesn't simply apply to making our ideal cut of toast. Particles in our body are normally

glycated constantly — wrinkles, waterfalls, coronary illness, and Alzheimer's Sickness are ramifications of glycation. It's a regular piece of maturing and keeping in mind that it can't be halted, it very well may be dialed back or accelerated.

The more glucose we convey to our body, the more frequently glycation occurs, and glycation's deliberate in an HbA1c test (the blood test for diabetes). The test estimates the number of red platelet proteins that have been glycated by glucose atoms in the former 3 months.

We put on weight,
When all the glucose our body needs for energy has been taken to the significant pieces of the body, it's fundamental that any abundance is removed from flow as quickly as time permits to lessen this free extreme creation and glycation.

Our body does this by utilizing three distinct inward stockpiling units. The liver transforms glucose into glycogen and here, it can cause no harm. The muscles can likewise store glucose as glycogen. Yet, we regularly eat substantially more glucose than we want, so these capacity units get full rapidly — which carries us to capacity unit number three Any overabundance of glucose that isn't put away as glycogen in our liver or muscles is transformed into fat. At whatever point the mitochondria in our cells need more energy, our body can turn the glycogen in the liver and muscles once again into glucose so it tends to be utilized. It's just when our glycogen stores decrease that we utilize our fat stores for energy — right now we're in fat-consuming mode, which is the point at which we get thinner.

The proviso here is that it's simply conceivable to consume fat assuming insulin levels are low one 2021 investigation discovered that weight reduction is constantly gone before by a decline in insulin levels. We've expounded on insulin and its job in glucose guidelines before however to put it plainly,

insulin assists lower with blooding sugar levels by empowering glucose to enter the phones. On the off chance that glucose levels increment, insulin is delivered. As glucose levels decline, insulin quits being delivered and its levels likewise decline. Thus, the steadier your glucose levels are, the steadier your

degrees of insulin will be, and your fat stores will have even more of an opportunity to fuel the body.

Wellbeing results of glucose spikes

The results of glucose spikes range from fleeting to those that stick around for a long stretch.

Is it true or not that you are worn out, as well?

One of the most widely recognized sensations of present-day life is that of sleepiness — this isn't the sluggishness we feel following a late evening or an exercise, but the baffling sensation of exhaustion despite doing everything we 'ought to' be accomplishing a solid way of life.

Indeed, it might shock no one that this feeling is likewise credited to glucose spikes. With rehashed glucose spikes, our mitochondria become full — they're straightforwardly loaded down with glucose and this

implies they're not able to change over glucose into energy effectively. Thus, the cells starve and as people, this is felt as sluggishness.

However, that is not all. Past this, glucose spikes can add to:

Steady appetite

Desires

Unfortunate rest

Colds

Hot flushes and night sweats

Skin inflammation

Issues with memory and focus

...also, that is simply temporary. Over the long run, steady glucose spikes have been displayed to add to additional serious inconveniences, for example,

Maturing and joint pain

Dementia and Alzheimer's Infection

Type 2 diabetes

Malignant growth risk Melancholy

Coronary illness

PCOS and fruitlessness

Non-alcoholic greasy liver

It's a major rundown we know. It's not there to unnerve you yet all things being equal, we trust it features exactly the way that significant glucose levels to your general wellbeing and prosperity.

Are some glucose spikes more regrettable than others?

We said before that all sugars separate into glucose. That implies that food like rice and pasta separate into glucose yet so does a cake or roll. The two of them cause glucose spikes however the sweet treat will be more awful for you for two reasons:

Chances are, the sweet treat has more sugar in it than the exquisite starch, so will cause a greater spike (and consequently a greater drop).

The sweet treat will contain sucrose, which contains fructose.

Glucose, sucrose, fructose — you could see they all end in - one and that is how you can realize they're all sugars. We've expounded on various kinds of sugar before however so, bland carbs like rice, pasta, and bread, all separate into glucose, while sweet sucrose separates into glucose and fructose.

All that in this article so far makes sense of what befalls glucose yet when we eat something sweet the body needs to likewise manage the fructose. Anyway, what occurs?

Indeed, not at all like glucose, fructose can't be transformed into glycogen and put away — the main thing that fructose can put away is fat. Fat from fructose will in general amass in the liver (high non-alcoholic greasy liver illness) in the middle between organs, as well as on the hips, thighs, and face. It additionally enters the circulatory system and adds to an expanded gamble of coronary illness.

It's hence that assuming two food sources have a similar number of calories, it's ideal to go for the exquisite choice. You'll in any case expand your glucose levels with glucose however without fructose, fewer atoms end up as fat. It's likewise worth staying alert that a great deal of sans-fat cycle food varieties contains sucrose, which as we presently realize separates into glucose and fructose, and fructose rises to fat. Keeping glucose levels stable

On the off chance that you have this far, well first and foremost — much obliged! Be that as it may, furthermore and above all, don't allow this data to get you down. Nothing in this article is planned to startle you into at absolutely no point ever eating a roll in the

future (as a matter of fact, you merit one for investing this energy perusing!). Thus, we will end on a high because while glucose spikes can cause all these short and long-haul confusions, decreasing these spikes (known as 'smoothing the glucose bend') can bring help. the food we eat may well have objective glucose spikes and their related issues, yet with little, basic changes we can utilize diet to keep glucose levels stable and our bodies cheerful.

There are one or two things you can do yet the following are three of the most straightforward ways of keeping your glucose levels stable — these work for the two individuals with and without type 2 diabetes. A paper distributed last year clarified that the best method for switching type 2 diabetes is to level our glucose bends.

Have an exquisite breakfast: what you have for breakfast can decide your desires and cravings for food until the end of the day, so consider trading your bowl of oat, for a flavorful choice like eggs to keep levels steadier.

Eat your vegetable initial: a new report demonstrated the way that eating your dinner in a specific request could decrease the glucose spike

after eating by however much 73% and the insulin spike by 48%. Examination into food requests is as yet progressing yet the proof in glucose the board is promising.

The reason is basic — whenever the situation allows, eat your vegetables first. This could mean eating the vegetables of your dish supper first or a side serving of mixed greens before eating a bowl of pasta. The thought is that the fiber of the vegetables covers the coating of the fascinating, which diminishes how much glucose is retained and how rapidly, prompting a steadier expansion in glucose as opposed to a spike.

Move after a feast: research proposes that a stroll after supper, frequently the greatest dinner of the day, can fundamentally lessen glucose levels for up to the following 24 hours. In any case, it doesn't need to be a walk — only 10 minutes of delicate development can assist with bringing down glucose levels as glucose is taken up by muscles for fuel.

The impact of glucose levels is shocking yet while there's a ton to take in, the main thing to detract from this is that with a complement glucose bend (less outrageous spikes and crashes), you can be useful for your physical and psychological wellness.

Chapter 3

How Might I Smooth My Glucose Bend

The degree of expansion in glucose in your blood after you eat and drink is a significant mark of metabolic well-being. It is typical for your blood glucose to ascend after you eat and afterward fall again as your body takes in the sugar from your blood to use for energy or to store. In any case, blood glucose levels that are ceaselessly too high are not great for us.

Concentrates on the show if we have any desire to oversee and keep a sound weight, we ought to focus on smoothing our post-feast glucose bends and not including calories. By straightening your blood glucose bends, you can consume more calories and lose more fat contrasted with individuals who eat fewer calories yet don't focus on leveling their glucose bends. Try not to have glucose spikes and your blood glucose bends will smooth.

At the point when we straighten our blood glucose bends, we enact a fountain of advantages including fewer desires, decreased hunger, and our time spent in fat-consuming mode is gotten to the next level.

The chemicals insulin and glucagon go about as an organization and are liable for keeping the blood glucose in a solid reach. At the point when blood glucose increments, insulin enacts the cells to take up sugar, and blood glucose is brought down. At the point when blood glucose drops excessively low; glucagon animates the arrival of glucose put away in the liver into the blood. Together they guarantee cells generally have sufficient energy to work.

Glucose is fundamental for our bodies as an energy source, and we have frameworks to process and store glucose for some time later. The liver and muscles are the essential stores (glucose put away as glycogen), and we can store around 15g of glycogen per kg body weight (around 1kg for a 70kg individual), and this is worked with by insulin.

The issue comes when we eat excessively or eat high GI food sources as the insulin additionally drives glucose into fat tissue (insulin doesn't especially store energy anyplace, however, 75% of the glucose carriers are in muscles, 25% in fat, and on the off chance that we are eating the perfect sum, the energy put away in fat tissue gets scorched). Sweet food varieties additionally contain fructose, which is handled by the liver, and when there are overabundance calories will be changed over and put away as fats as opposed to being switched over completely to glucose (which occurs if you're not gorging sugar/fructose).

At the point when blood glucose is constantly high our insulin levels are persistently raised and getting more fit turns out to be a lot harder. At the point when we decline our blood glucose level, our insulin levels drop as well, and insulin decrease is fundamental and consistently goes before weight loss3. If we don't hold our insulin under tight restraints, we move into fat capacity mode rather than fat-consuming mode.

Figuring out how to adjust your glucose and balance out post-feast blood glucose spikes can be simple and manageable with the right help setup. Utilizing the accompanying instruments will uphold a sound glucose and insulin reaction.

You might have the option to assist with keeping your glucose stable by making changes to your eating regimen, including diminishing sugar and refined carbs, drinking sufficient water, and getting customary activity.

1. Go low-carb

Starches (carbs) cause glucose to rise.
At the point when you eat carbs, they are separated into straightforward sugars. Those sugars then enter the circulation system.

As your glucose levels rise, your pancreas delivers a chemical called insulin, which prompts your phones to retain sugar from the blood. This causes your glucose levels to drop. Many examinations have shown that consuming a low-carb diet can assist with forestalling glucose spikes

Low-carb counts calories additionally have the additional advantage of helping weight reduction, which can likewise diminish glucose spikes.
There are heaps of ways of decreasing your carb admission, including counting carbs. This is an aide while heading to make it happen.

2. Eat less refined carbs

Refined carbs, also called handled carbs, are sugars or refined grains.
A few normal wellsprings of refined carbs are table sugar, white bread, white rice, pop, sweets, breakfast oats, and pastries.

Refined carbs have been deprived of practically all supplements, nutrients, minerals, and fiber.

Refined carbs are said to have a high glycemic profile since they are effectively and immediately processed by the body. This prompts glucose spikes. An enormous observational investigation of more than 91,000 ladies

found that an eating routine high in high-glycemic-file carbs was related to an expansion in type 2 diabetes The spike in glucose and ensuing drop you might insight after eating high-glycemic-file food sources can likewise advance appetite and can prompt gorging and weight gain.

The glycemic list of carbs differs. It's impacted by various things, including readiness, what else you eat, and how the carbs are cooked or ready.

By and large, entire grain food sources have a lower glycemic record, as do most organic products, non-bland vegetables, and vegetables.

3. Diminish your sugar admission

The typical American consumes 22 teaspoons (88 grams) of added sugar each day. That means around 350 calories.

While a portion of this is added as table sugar, its vast majority comes from handled and arranged food sources, like treats, treats, and soft drinks.
You have no healthful requirement for added sugar like sucrose and high-fructose corn syrup. They are essentially, simply void of calories.

Your body separates these straightforward sugars effectively, causing a practically quick spike in glucose. Concentrates on showing that consuming sugars are related to creating insulin obstruction.

This is the point at which the cells neglect to answer as they ought to the arrival of insulin, bringing about the body not having the option to control glucose really
In 2016, the US Food and Medication Organization (FDA) meaningfully impacted how food sources must be marked in the US. Food varieties currently need to show how much-added sugars they contain in grams and as a level of the suggested everyday greatest admission.

An elective choice to surrender sugar altogether is to supplant it with sugar substitutes.

4. Keep a sound weight

As of now, two out of three grown-ups in the US are viewed as overweight or hefty Being overweight or hefty can make it harder for your body to utilize insulin and control glucose levels. This can prompt glucose spikes and a comparing higher gamble of creating type 2 diabetes. The exact ways it works are as yet muddled, yet there's heaps of proof connecting heftiness to insulin opposition and the advancement of type 2 diabetes Weight reduction, then again, has been displayed to further develop glucose control.

In one review, 35 hefty individuals lost a normal of 14.5 pounds (6.6 kg) north of 12 weeks while they were on a careful nutritional plan of 1,600 calories per day. Their glucose dropped by a normal of 14%
In one more investigation of individuals without diabetes, weight reduction was found to diminish the frequency of creating type 2 diabetes by 58%

5. Practice more

The practice assists control of blood sugar spikes by expanding the responsiveness of your cells to the chemical insulin.

Practice additionally makes muscle cells assimilate sugar from the blood, assisting with bringing down glucose levels. Both focused energy and

moderate-power practices have been found to diminish glucose spikes.
One review found comparable enhancements in glucose control in 27 grown-ups who completed either medium- or focused energy workouts.

Whether you practice on a vacant or full stomach could affect glucose control. One review found practice performed before breakfast controlled glucose more really than practice done after breakfast.
Expanding exercise likewise has the additional advantage of assisting with weight reduction, a one-two punch to battle glucose spikes

6. Eat more fiber

Fiber is comprised of pieces of plant food that your body can't process. It is frequently separated into two gatherings: dissolvable and insoluble fiber. Solvent fiber, specifically, can assist with controlling glucose spikes.

It breaks down in the water to shape a gel-like substance that eases back the retention of carbs in the stomach.

This outcome is a consistent ascent and falls in glucose, as opposed to a spike.

Fiber can likewise encourage you, lessening your hunger and food consumption.
Great wellsprings of solvent fiber include: Oats
Nuts
Vegetables
A few organic products, like apples, oranges, and blueberries
Numerous vegetables

7. Hydrate

Not drinking sufficient water can prompt glucose spikes. At the point when you are got dried out, your body delivers a chemical called vasopressin. This urges your kidneys to hold liquid and prevent the body from flushing out the overabundance of sugar in your pee. It additionally prompts your liver to deliver more sugar into the blood

One investigation of 3,615 individuals found that the people who drank no less than 34 ounces (around 1 liter) of water a day were 21% less inclined to foster high glucose than the people who drank 16 ounces (473 ml) or less a day.

A drawn-out concentrate on 4,742 individuals in Sweden found that, over 12.6 years, an increment of vasopressin in the blood was connected to an expansion in insulin obstruction and type 2 diabetes.

How much water you ought to drink is frequently up for conversation. It relies upon the person. Continuously ensure you drink when you're parched and increment your water consumption during blistering climates or while working out. Stick to water instead of sweet squeeze or soft drinks, since the sugar content will prompt glucose spikes.

8. Bring some vinegar into your eating routine

Vinegar, especially apple juice vinegar, has been found to have numerous medical advantages.
It has been connected to weight reduction, cholesterol decrease, antibacterial properties, and glucose control,
A few investigations demonstrate the way that

consuming vinegar can increment insulin reaction and diminish glucose spikes

One review found vinegar essentially diminished glucose in members who had recently consumed a dinner containing 50 grams of carbs. The investigation likewise discovered that the more grounded the vinegar, the lower the glucose.

One more review investigated the impact of vinegar on glucose after members consumed carbs. It found that vinegar expanded insulin

responsiveness by somewhere in the range of 19% and 34%.

The expansion of vinegar can likewise bring down the glycemic record of food, which can assist with diminishing glucose spikes.

A concentrate in Japan found that adding salted food varieties to rice diminished the glycemic file of the dinner fundamentally

9. Bring some vinegar into your eating regimen

Vinegar, especially apple juice vinegar, has been found to have numerous medical advantages. It has been connected to weight reduction, cholesterol decrease, antibacterial properties, and glucose control.

A few examinations demonstrate the way that consuming vinegar can increment insulin reaction and lessen glucose spikes.

One review found vinegar essentially diminished glucose in members who had recently consumed a feast containing 50 grams of carbs. The investigation likewise discovered that the more grounded the vinegar, the lower the glucose.

One more review investigated the impact of vinegar on glucose after members consumed carbs. It found that vinegar expanded insulin awareness by somewhere in the range of 19% and 34%. The expansion of vinegar can likewise bring down the glycemic record of food, which can assist with diminishing glucose spikes.

A concentrate in Japan found that adding salted food varieties to rice diminished the glycemic file of the dinner fundamentally

10. Get sufficient chromium and magnesium
Concentrates show both chromium and magnesium can be viable in controlling glucose spikes.

Chromium

Chromium is a mineral that you want in limited quantities.

Upgrading the activity of insulin is thought. This could assist with controlling glucose spikes by empowering the phones to assimilate sugar from the blood.
In one little review, 13 solid men were given 75 grams of white bread regardless of chromium added. The expansion of chromium brought about a 20% decrease in glucose following the dinner.

Suggested dietary admissions for chromium can be tracked down hereTrusted Source. Rich food sources incorporate broccoli, egg yolks, shellfish, tomatoes, and Brazil nuts.

Magnesium

Magnesium is one more mineral that has been connected to glucose control.

In one investigation of 48 individuals, half were given a 600-mg magnesium supplement alongside way-of-life counsel, while the other half were simply offered way-of-life guidance. Insulin responsiveness expanded in the gathering given magnesium supplements.

Another review explored the joint impacts of enhancing chromium and magnesium on glucose. They tracked down that a mix of the two expanded insulin responsiveness more than either supplement alone. Suggested dietary admissions for magnesium can be tracked down hereTrusted Source. Rich food sources incorporate spinach, almonds, avocados, cashews, and peanuts.

11. Brighten up your life

Cinnamon and fenugreek have been utilized in elective medication for millennia. They have both been connected to glucose control.

Cinnamon

The logical proof for the utilization of cinnamon in glucose control is blended.

In solid individuals, cinnamon has been displayed to increment insulin responsiveness and lessen glucose spikes following a carb-based dinner.

One of these investigations followed 14 solid individuals.

It found that eating 6 grams of cinnamon with 300 grams of rice pudding essentially diminished glucose spikes, contrasted with eating the pudding alone. In any case, there are likewise concentrates that show cinnamon meaningfully affects glucose.

One survey took a gander at 10 excellent examinations in a sum of 577 individuals with diabetes. The audit found no huge distinction in glucose spikes after members had taken cinnamon.

There are two kinds of cinnamon:

Cassia: Can emerge out of a few unique types of Cinnamomum trees. This is the sort most ordinarily tracked down in many grocery stores.

Ceylon: Comes explicitly from the Cinnamomum verum tree. It is more costly, yet may contain more cell reinforcements.

Cassia cinnamon contains a possibly destructive substance called coumarin.

The European Food Handling Authority (EFSA) has set the average day-to-day admission of coumarin at 0.045 mg per pound of body weight (0.1mg/kg). This is around a portion of a teaspoon (1 gram) of Cassia cinnamon for a 165-pound (75-kg) individual.

Fenugreek

One of the properties of fenugreek is that the seeds are high in solvent fiber. This forestalls glucose spikes by dialing back the assimilation and ingestion of carbs.

Notwithstanding, apparently glucose levels might profit from something other than the seeds.

An examination of 10 investigations discovered that fenugreek altogether decreased glucose two hours after eating.

Fenugreek might assist with lessening glucose spikes. It tends to be added to food, however, it has a seriously solid taste, so certain individuals like to accept it as an enhancement

12. Attempt berberine

Berberine is a substance that can be separated from a few distinct plants. It has been utilized in conventional Chinese medication for millennia. A portion of its purposes incorporates cholesterol decrease, weight reduction, and glucose control. Berberine decreases how much sugar is delivered by the liver and increments insulin awareness. It has even been viewed as successful as certain

medications utilized for type 2 diabetes.

One review took a gander at 116 individuals with type 2 diabetes who either got berberine or a fake treatment for a very long time. Berberine diminished glucose spikes after dinner by 25%. Notwithstanding, another review found berberine caused secondary effects in certain individuals, like loose bowels, obstruction, and gas. Although berberine seems, by all accounts, to be genuinely protected, address your PCP before taking it assuming you have any ailments or are taking any drug.

13. Consider this way of life factors

If you truly have any desire to decrease your glucose spikes, you ought to likewise consider this way of life factors that can influence glucose.

Stress

Stress can adversely influence your well-being in various ways, causing cerebral pains, expanded circulatory strain, and tension.

It has additionally been displayed to influence glucose. As feelings of anxiety go up, your body delivers specific chemicals. The impact is to deliver put away energy as sugar into your circulatory system for the instinctive reaction.

One investigation of 241 Italian laborers found an expansion in business-related pressure was straightforwardly connected to an expansion in glucose levels.

Effectively addressing pressure has additionally been found to help your glucose. In an investigation of nursing understudies, yoga practices were found to decrease pressure and glucose spikes following a feast.

Rest
Both excessively little and a lot of rest have been related to unfortunate glucose control.
In any event, having a couple of terrible evenings can influence your glucose levels.

An investigation of nine sound individuals showed that resting pretty much nothing, or just for 4 hours, expanded insulin obstruction and glucose levels. With rest, quality is pretty much as significant as the amount. A review viewed the most profound degree of rest as most significant as far as controlling glucose.

Liquor
Cocktails frequently contain a great deal of added sugar. This is especially valid for blended beverages and mixed drinks, which can contain as much as 30 grams of sugar for every serving.
The sugar in cocktails will cause glucose spikes similar to added sugar in food. Most cocktails additionally have practically no dietary benefit.

Likewise, with added sugar, they are unfilled calories. Besides, over the long run, weighty drinking can diminish the adequacy of insulin, which prompts high glucose and can ultimately prompt sort 2 diabetes.
In any case, concentrates on demonstrating the way that moderate, controlled drinking can really have a defensive impact concerning glucose control and can likewise bring down the gamble of creating type 2 diabetes. One investigation discovered that drinking moderate measures of liquor with feast might diminish glucose spikes by up to 37%

Conclusion

In the previous ten years, the quantity of individuals in the U.S. who have been impacted by diabetes has developed at a fast rate. The most widely recognized event of diabetes will be diabetes mellitus (DM). On the off chance that you're determined to have DM, checking your blood glucose is a key stage in dealing with this medical issue. Work with your medical care group so you stay inside the blood glucose target they set for you. The better your blood glucose is controlled, the better you will be

www.ingramcontent.com/pod-product-compliance
Lightning Source LLC
Chambersburg PA
CBHW061532250726
48657CB00005B/2202